PREPPER'S SURVIVAL NATURAL MEDICINE:

An Ultimate Guide Needed When There's no Medical Personnel, Acute Knowledge About First Aid, Life-saving Herbs, and Natural Remedies

BY

CHRISTOPHER DEVINE

TABLE OF CONTENTS

INTRODUCTION

In an ever-changing world where uncertainties loom on the horizon, a growing community of individuals is embracing the ethos of self-reliance and preparedness. As we navigate through the complexities of modern life, the concept of prepping has gained traction, encouraging people to equip themselves with the skills and resources necessary to thrive in the face of unforeseen challenges. One pivotal aspect of this preparedness movement is the exploration of natural medicine as an integral component of prepper survival strategies.

Preppers, individuals dedicated to readiness for any disruptive event, whether natural disasters, economic instability, or societal unrest, understand the importance of holistic well-being. While traditional medical practices have undoubtedly played a vital role in human health, an increasing number of preppers are turning to the age-old wisdom of natural medicine to complement their preparedness efforts. This approach, rooted in the use of medicinal plants, herbs, and alternative therapies, offers a time-tested and often sustainable means of addressing health concerns when conventional resources may be limited or inaccessible.

In this exploration of Prepper's Survival Natural Medicine, we delve into the rich tapestry of botanical remedies, ancestral healing practices, and the profound knowledge that has been passed down through generations. As we journey through the annals of herbalism, we uncover the potent potential of nature's pharmacy, discovering how preppers are integrating these natural remedies into their survival toolkits.

This comprehensive guide aims to shed light on the principles of natural medicine, exploring the medicinal properties of plants that have been cherished for centuries. From the meticulous preparation of herbal tinctures to the cultivation of healing gardens, preppers are rekindling a profound connection with the Earth as they prepare for uncertain times. As we unravel the pages of this exploration, we'll examine the practical applications of natural medicine in various survival scenarios, empowering preppers to fortify their health and resilience in the face of adversity.

In the following chapters, we will traverse the realms of herbal lore, traditional healing systems, and the invaluable knowledge that empowers individuals to become stewards of their well-being. Whether it's harnessing the anti-inflammatory properties of turmeric, the immune-boosting capabilities of echinacea, or the calming effects of chamomile, each botanical ally becomes a testament to the prepper's commitment to self-sufficiency.

Join us on this enlightening journey into the realm of Prepper's Survival Natural Medicine, where the synergy between nature and preparedness becomes a beacon of resilience in an unpredictable world. As we unlock the secrets of plant-based healing, we embark on a transformative exploration of self-sufficiency, sustainability, and the timeless wisdom encoded in the natural remedies that have stood the test of time.

CHAPTER 1: FOUNDATIONS OF EMERGENCY PREPAREDNESS

Understanding the Prepper Mindset

In an unpredictable world, being prepared for emergencies is not just a prudent choice but a necessity. The foundations of emergency preparedness go beyond stockpiling supplies and creating evacuation plans; they delve into the mindset of preppers - individuals who proactively equip themselves to handle unforeseen challenges. Understanding the prepper mindset is crucial for cultivating a resilient and self-reliant approach to emergency preparedness.

Risk Awareness:

Preppers exhibit a heightened awareness of potential risks and threats, whether natural disasters, economic downturns, or societal unrest. This mindset involves a commitment to staying informed about global events, assessing local vulnerabilities, and recognizing the potential impact on one's community and personal life.

Self-Reliance:

At the core of the prepper mindset is the belief in self-reliance. Preppers understand that relying solely on external aid during emergencies may not be sufficient. They strive to develop the skills and resources needed to sustain themselves and their families independently for an extended period.

Strategic Planning:

Preppers engage in strategic planning that extends beyond mere survival. They create comprehensive emergency plans, considering factors like food and water storage, alternative energy sources, medical supplies, and communication strategies. This planning involves a holistic approach to addressing various aspects of life during and after an emergency.

Skill Acquisition:

Beyond stockpiling physical resources, preppers invest time and effort in acquiring a diverse set of skills. From first aid and basic survival skills to gardening, hunting, and DIY repairs, preppers recognize the value of being versatile in facing unforeseen challenges.

Community Building:

Contrary to the stereotype of preppers as isolated individuals, many actively engage in community building. The prepper mindset recognizes the strength that comes from collaboration and mutual support. This involves sharing knowledge, resources, and skills within a community to enhance overall resilience.

Adaptability:

Preppers understand the importance of adaptability in the face of evolving situations. The ability to adjust plans, strategies, and expectations is a key aspect of the prepper mindset. Flexibility allows preppers to navigate unpredictable circumstances with resilience and effectiveness.

Long-Term Sustainability:

Preppers look beyond short-term survival and focus on long-term sustainability. This involves considerations such as renewable energy sources, sustainable food production, and conservation practices. The prepper mindset acknowledges the interconnectedness of environmental, economic, and social factors in building a resilient future.

Mindset of Continual Improvement:

The prepper mindset is not static; it is a mindset of continual improvement. Preppers regularly assess their plans, update their skill sets, and adapt to changing circumstances. This commitment to ongoing improvement ensures that preppers remain effective and adaptable in the face of evolving challenges.

The foundations of emergency preparedness lie in understanding and adopting the prepper mindset. By embracing risk awareness, self-reliance, strategic planning, skill acquisition, community building, adaptability, long-term sustainability, and a mindset of continual improvement, individuals can better equip themselves to face the uncertainties of the future. Ultimately, the prepper mindset is not just about surviving emergencies; it's about thriving in the midst of adversity and building a more resilient and self-sufficient community.

Building a Basic Emergency Kit

In an unpredictable world, being prepared for emergencies is crucial to ensuring the safety and well-being of ourselves and our loved ones. One fundamental aspect of emergency preparedness is the creation of a basic emergency kit. This kit serves as a lifeline during unexpected situations, providing essential items to sustain you and your family until help arrives. In this guide, we will explore the foundations of emergency preparedness and walk you through the process of building a basic emergency kit.

Understanding the Risks:

Before assembling your emergency kit, it's important to assess the potential risks in your area. Different regions face various natural disasters such as earthquakes, hurricanes, floods, wildfires, or severe storms. Identify the specific risks in your locality to tailor your emergency kit accordingly.

Water and Hydration:

Water is a fundamental necessity for survival. In your emergency kit, include at least one gallon of water per person per day for a minimum of three days. Ensure you have enough water for both drinking and sanitation purposes. Consider portable water purification tablets or filters for an added layer of security.

Non-Perishable Food:

Include a supply of non-perishable food items that require little to no preparation. Examples include canned goods, energy bars, dried fruits, nuts, and other high-calorie snacks. Aim for a three-day supply for each person in your household.

First Aid Kit:

A well-equipped first aid kit is essential for handling injuries and medical emergencies. Your kit should include bandages, antiseptic wipes, pain relievers, adhesive tape, scissors, tweezers, and any necessary prescription medications. Regularly check and update your first aid supplies to ensure they remain current.

Clothing and Personal Items:

Pack a set of sturdy clothing, including comfortable shoes, for each family member.

Consider the climate in your area and any specific needs, such as rain gear or cold-weather clothing. Don't forget personal items such as hygiene products, prescription eyewear, and important documents stored in a waterproof container.

Lighting and Communication:

Include a flashlight with extra batteries or, ideally, a hand-crank or solar-powered flashlight. A battery-operated or hand-crank radio is also crucial for receiving emergency alerts and information. Consider adding a whistle to your kit for signaling purposes.

Shelter and Warmth:

In case you need to evacuate or find temporary shelter, pack a lightweight and durable emergency tent or tarp. Include sleeping bags or blankets for each family member to provide warmth during colder conditions.

Tools and Multipurpose Items:
Include a multi-tool, duct tape, and basic tools such as pliers and a wrench. These items can be invaluable for quick repairs or improvisations during emergencies.

Building a basic emergency kit is a foundational step in preparing for unforeseen circumstances. Regularly review and update your kit to ensure its effectiveness. By taking these essential measures, you empower yourself and your family to face emergencies with confidence and resilience. Remember, preparedness is key, and a well-assembled emergency kit can make all the difference when it matters most.

Developing a Family Emergency Plan

In an unpredictable world, being prepared for emergencies is a crucial aspect of ensuring the safety and well-being of your family. Whether it's a natural disaster, a power outage, or a sudden evacuation, having a well-thought-out Family Emergency Plan is the cornerstone of effective emergency preparedness. This guide will walk you through the essential steps to develop a comprehensive plan that will empower your family to face unexpected challenges with confidence.

Step 1: Risk Assessment

Begin by identifying potential risks in your area. Consider natural disasters such as earthquakes, floods, hurricanes, or wildfires, as well as man-made emergencies like power outages, industrial accidents, or civil unrest. Understanding the specific threats in your region will help tailor your emergency plan to address those unique challenges.

Step 2: Communication Strategy

Establishing effective communication channels is paramount during emergencies. Create a list of emergency contacts, including family members, neighbors, and friends. Ensure everyone knows how to reach each other and designate an out-of-town contact person, as local lines may be congested during a crisis. Familiarize yourself with emergency alert systems and subscribe to local alerts to stay informed about potential threats.

Step 3: Evacuation Plan

Develop a detailed evacuation plan that includes multiple routes and meeting points. Identify safe locations both within your home and in your community. Consider the needs of all family members, including pets, elderly relatives, or individuals with special medical requirements. Practice evacuation drills regularly to ensure everyone is familiar with the procedures.

Step 4: Emergency Kit

Prepare a well-stocked emergency kit that can sustain your family for at least 72 hours. Include essentials such as water, non-perishable food, medications, first aid supplies, flashlights, batteries, important documents, cash, and personal hygiene items. Tailor the kit to meet the specific needs of your family members, such as baby supplies, pet food, or medical equipment.

Step 5: Medical Information

Compile a list of medical information for each family member, including allergies, current medications, and emergency contacts. Keep copies of important documents like insurance cards, identification, and medical records in a waterproof container as part of your emergency kit.

Step 6: Training and Education

Ensure that every family member is familiar with basic emergency procedures. Teach children how to call emergency services and explain the importance of following evacuation routes. Consider taking first aid and CPR courses as a family, and regularly review and update your emergency plan to reflect any changes in your family's circumstances.

Step 7: Regular Review and Update

Emergency plans should be living documents that adapt to the evolving needs of your family and changes in your community. Conduct regular reviews and updates, especially after experiencing a significant event or if there are alterations in family dynamics, health conditions, or living arrangements.

By taking the time to develop a comprehensive Family Emergency Plan, you are taking a proactive approach to safeguarding your loved ones during challenging times. Remember, preparedness is the key to resilience. Be ready, stay informed, and empower your family to face emergencies with confidence and cohesion.

CHAPTER 2: FIRST AID ESSENTIALS

Assessing and Treating Common Injuries

Accidents can happen anytime, anywhere, and having a basic understanding of first aid essentials is crucial. Knowing how to assess and treat common injuries can make a significant difference in minimizing damage and potentially saving lives. In this guide, we'll explore key first aid principles for assessing and treating common injuries.

I. Initial Assessment:

A. Scene Safety:

Ensure your safety and the safety of others before approaching the scene.

Identify potential hazards and take necessary precautions.

Call for professional help if needed.

B. Primary Survey:

Check for responsiveness: Tap the person and ask if they are okay.

Assess the person's airway, breathing, and circulation (ABC).

Provide basic life support if necessary (CPR).

II. Treating Common Injuries:

A. Cuts and Scrapes:

Clean the wound with mild soap and water.

Apply an antiseptic ointment to prevent infection.

Cover the wound with a sterile dressing or bandage.

B. Burns:

For minor burns, run cool water over the affected area for at least 10 minutes.

Do not use ice or very cold water.

Cover the burn with a clean, non-stick bandage.

C. Fractures and Sprains:

Immobilize the injured area with a splint if possible.

Apply a cold compress to reduce swelling.

Seek professional medical attention for proper diagnosis and treatment.

D. Choking:

Encourage the person to cough forcefully.

Perform abdominal thrusts (Heimlich maneuver) if the person is unable to breathe.

Call for emergency assistance if the obstruction persists.

E. Head Injuries:

Keep the person still and call for professional help.

Apply a cold compress to reduce swelling.

Monitor for signs of concussion or altered consciousness.

F. Nosebleeds:

Have the person lean forward and pinch the nostrils together.

Apply pressure for at least 10 minutes.

Avoid tilting the head backward to prevent blood from flowing into the throat.

III. Additional Tips:

A. Maintain First Aid Supplies:

Keep a well-stocked first aid kit at home, in the car, and at work.

Regularly check and replenish supplies to ensure readiness.

B. Stay Informed:

Attend first aid training courses to enhance your skills.

Stay updated on the latest first aid guidelines and techniques.

Being equipped with first aid essentials and knowing how to assess and treat common injuries empowers individuals to act swiftly in emergency situations. By following these guidelines, you can make a positive impact during critical moments and contribute to the well-being of those around you. Remember, quick and informed actions can make a significant difference in the outcomes of accidents and injuries.

Basic Life Support Techniques

First aid is a crucial skill that everyone should possess, as it can make a significant difference in emergencies. Basic life support (BLS) techniques are fundamental components of first aid, designed to sustain life until professional medical help arrives. In this guide, we will explore essential first aid techniques that can be the difference between life and death in critical situations.

Check for Safety:

Before approaching the scene, ensure your safety and the safety of others.

Assess potential hazards such as traffic, fire, or dangerous substances.

Assess the Situation:

Evaluate the individual's responsiveness by gently tapping and shouting.

Call for emergency help immediately if the person is unresponsive.

Open the Airway:

Place the person on their back on a firm surface.

Tilt their head backward and lift the chin to open the airway.

Check for Breathing:

Look, listen, and feel for breathing.

If not breathing, start rescue breaths.

Perform CPR (Cardiopulmonary Resuscitation):

If the person is not breathing and has no pulse, initiate CPR.

Administer chest compressions at a rate of 100-120 compressions per minute.

Follow the recommended compression-to-ventilation ratio.

Use an AED (Automated External Defibrillator):

If available, use an AED to analyze the heart's rhythm and deliver a shock if necessary.

Follow the AED's prompts and continue CPR until professional help arrives.

Control Bleeding:

Apply direct pressure to the wound using a sterile dressing or clean cloth.

Elevate the injured limb if possible and maintain pressure until bleeding stops.

Treat Shock:

Keep the person warm by covering them with a blanket.

Elevate the legs unless there are signs of head, neck, or back injury.

Assist with Choking:

If the person is conscious, encourage coughing.

If choking persists, perform abdominal thrusts (Heimlich maneuver) until the object is expelled.

Manage Burns:

Cool the burn with running cold water for at least 10 minutes.

Cover the burn with a sterile non-stick dressing.

Attend to Fractures and Sprains:
Immobilize the injured area with a splint.
Apply ice to reduce swelling, and seek medical help.
Being equipped with basic life support techniques is essential for anyone, as emergencies can happen at any time. By staying calm, assessing the situation, and applying these first aid essentials, you can provide crucial assistance until professional help arrives. Consider taking a first aid and CPR course to enhance your skills and confidence in handling emergency situations. Remember, your quick and effective response can save lives.

Handling Medical Emergencies Without Professional Help

In times of medical emergencies, the ability to provide immediate and effective first aid can make a crucial difference in saving lives and preventing further harm. While professional help is essential, there are instances where immediate action is required before medical professionals arrive. This emphasizes the importance of having a basic understanding of first aid essentials. In this guide, we will explore key first aid principles and techniques that can empower individuals to respond confidently in various emergency situations.

Assessment and Prioritization:

Begin by assessing the situation for potential dangers to yourself and others.

Prioritize the needs of the injured, focusing on life-threatening conditions such as severe bleeding, difficulty breathing, or unconsciousness.

Emergency Contact:

Call emergency services immediately. Provide accurate information about the situation, location, and the number of individuals involved.

Stay on the line and follow the dispatcher's instructions.

CPR (Cardiopulmonary Resuscitation):

Learn and practice CPR techniques for adults, children, and infants.

Understand the importance of early CPR to maintain blood circulation and oxygen supply until professional help arrives.

Choking:

Recognize the signs of choking and intervene promptly.

Perform the Heimlich maneuver for adults and children, adjusting the force based on the individual's age.

Bleeding and Wound Care:

Control bleeding by applying direct pressure to the wound using a clean cloth or bandage.

Elevate the injured area if possible and maintain pressure until bleeding stops or professional help arrives.

Shock Management:

Recognize the symptoms of shock, such as pale skin, rapid breathing, and confusion.

Keep the individual warm and comfortable, laying them down with their legs elevated slightly if no spinal injury is suspected.

Burns:

Cool burns with running water for at least 10 minutes.

Cover the burn with a clean, non-stick bandage.

Fractures and Sprains:

Immobilize the injured limb to prevent further damage.

Apply ice to reduce swelling and elevate the limb if possible.

Seizures:

Create a safe space by removing nearby objects.

Do not restrain the individual during a seizure; instead, protect them from potential hazards.

Allergic Reactions:

Administer an epinephrine auto-injector (if available) for severe allergic reactions.

Call for emergency medical assistance immediately.

Being prepared to handle medical emergencies without professional help is a valuable skill that can make a significant impact in critical situations. Regularly updating your knowledge of first aid essentials and participating in relevant training courses can enhance your ability to respond effectively when it matters most. Remember, quick and informed action can be the key to saving lives and minimizing the impact of medical emergencies.

CHAPTER 3:
LIFE-SAVING HERBS
FOR SURVIVAL

Creating Herbal Remedies for Common Ailments

In a world where modern medicine may not always be readily available, knowing how to utilize nature's pharmacy becomes a valuable skill. Herbs have been used for centuries for their medicinal properties, and in survival situations, they can be crucial for treating common ailments. This guide explores life-saving herbs and how to create herbal remedies for various health issues.

Aloe Vera:

Benefits: Aloe Vera is renowned for its healing properties, particularly for burns, cuts, and skin irritations.

Herbal Remedy: Break open an Aloe Vera leaf and apply the gel directly to burns or wounds for soothing relief.

Chamomile:

Benefits: Chamomile has calming and anti-inflammatory properties, making it effective for stress relief and digestive issues.

Herbal Remedy: Make a chamomile tea by steeping dried flowers in hot water. This can help alleviate anxiety and indigestion.

Echinacea:

Benefits: Known for its immune-boosting properties, Echinacea can help prevent and alleviate symptoms of the common cold.

Herbal Remedy: Brew Echinacea tea or create a tincture using the plant's roots and leaves.

Garlic:

Benefits: Garlic is a potent antibacterial and antiviral herb that can help fight infections and boost overall immune function.

Herbal Remedy: Consume raw garlic or make a garlic-infused oil for treating respiratory issues.

Ginger:

Benefits: Ginger is anti-inflammatory and aids digestion, making it valuable for relieving nausea, motion sickness, and muscle pain.

Herbal Remedy: Prepare ginger tea or chew on raw ginger to combat nausea and promote digestion.

Lavender:

Benefits: Lavender is known for its calming effects, making it an excellent remedy for stress, anxiety, and sleep disorders.

Herbal Remedy: Use lavender essential oil in a diffuser or apply diluted oil to the skin for relaxation.

Peppermint:

Benefits: Peppermint has digestive benefits and can also relieve headaches and muscle pain.

Herbal Remedy: Brew peppermint tea or apply diluted peppermint oil to the temples for headache relief.

Calendula:

Benefits: Calendula possesses anti-inflammatory and antifungal properties, making it useful for skin issues like cuts and rashes.

Herbal Remedy: Create a salve using calendula-infused oil for topical application on minor skin irritations.

Turmeric:

Benefits: Turmeric is a powerful anti-inflammatory and antioxidant herb that can aid in relieving joint pain and inflammation.

Herbal Remedy: Make a turmeric paste by mixing the powdered herb with water and apply it to affected areas.

Thyme:

Benefits: Thyme has antimicrobial properties, making it beneficial for respiratory infections and coughs.

Herbal Remedy: Prepare thyme tea or use thyme-infused honey for soothing respiratory discomfort.

In a survival scenario, knowing how to identify, harvest, and utilize life-saving herbs can be a valuable skill. While these remedies can provide relief for common ailments, it's essential to seek professional medical help for serious health issues. Building a knowledge base on herbal remedies empowers individuals to take control of their health and well-being, especially when conventional medical resources may be limited.

Understanding the Healing Properties of Herbs

In the realm of survival, the ability to harness the healing power of nature is a skill that can be the difference between life and death. Throughout history, various cultures have turned to herbs for their medicinal properties, relying on the wisdom of nature to address a myriad of health concerns. In the context of survival, knowing which herbs can be life-saving is crucial. This article explores the healing properties of certain herbs that could prove invaluable in a survival situation.

Aloe Vera: The Desert's First Aid Plant

Aloe vera, with its fleshy leaves, is a well-known succulent revered for its soothing properties. In survival scenarios, the gel inside its leaves can be applied topically to treat burns, wounds, and skin irritations. Aloe vera's anti-inflammatory and antimicrobial qualities make it a natural first aid remedy.

Echinacea: Nature's Immune Booster

Echinacea, also known as the purple coneflower, has been used by Native Americans for centuries to bolster the immune system. This herb is believed to reduce the severity and duration of colds and flu. In a survival situation, maintaining a strong immune system is essential, and echinacea can be a valuable ally.

Garlic: Nature's Antibiotic

Garlic, renowned for its culinary uses, also possesses potent medicinal properties. Allicin, a compound found in garlic, has natural antibiotic and antiviral effects. In survival situations where access to modern medicine is limited, garlic can be consumed to help combat infections and boost overall health.

Calendula: The Skin Healer

Calendula, or pot marigold, is known for its skin-healing properties. It has anti-inflammatory and antiseptic qualities, making it effective for treating wounds, cuts, and skin infections. Calendula can be used topically as a poultice or infused into a salve for its healing benefits.

Chamomile: Nature's Calming Agent

Chamomile, often enjoyed as a soothing tea, has calming and anti-anxiety properties. In survival situations where stress levels can be high, chamomile can help promote relaxation and better sleep. Additionally, its anti-inflammatory properties make it beneficial for treating digestive issues.

Turmeric: The Anti-Inflammatory Powerhouse

Turmeric, with its active compound curcumin, is a potent anti-inflammatory and antioxidant herb. In survival situations where injuries and inflammation are common, turmeric can be consumed to aid in reducing pain and promoting healing.

St. John's Wort: Nature's Antidepressant

St. John's Wort is known for its mood-enhancing properties. In a survival scenario where mental well-being is crucial, this herb can be used to alleviate symptoms of mild to moderate depression and anxiety.

Understanding the healing properties of herbs is a valuable skill for survivalists and outdoor enthusiasts alike. While these herbs can offer natural remedies, it's essential to educate oneself thoroughly and, when possible, consult with a healthcare professional. In a survival situation, the knowledge of life-saving herbs can be the key to overcoming health challenges when conventional medical assistance is not readily available. Nature's pharmacy provides a wealth of resources; it's up to us to unlock their potential for the sake of our well-being in challenging circumstances.

CHAPTER 4:
NATURAL REMEDIES
FOR COMMON
CONDITIONS

Addressing Pain and Inflammation Naturally

Pain and inflammation are common discomforts that affect millions of people worldwide. While conventional medications can provide relief, many individuals seek alternative, natural remedies to manage these conditions. In this article, we'll explore some natural remedies that have been traditionally used to address pain and inflammation.

Turmeric:

Active Ingredient: Curcumin, the main active compound in turmeric, has powerful anti-inflammatory and antioxidant properties.

Usage: Incorporate turmeric into your diet through curries, teas, or supplements.

Benefits: Studies suggest that turmeric may help alleviate symptoms of arthritis, joint pain, and inflammation.

Ginger:

Active Compounds: Gingerol and zingerone contribute to ginger's anti-inflammatory effects.

Usage: Consume fresh ginger in tea, add it to meals, or take ginger supplements.

Benefits: Ginger is known for its ability to reduce muscle pain, osteoarthritis symptoms, and menstrual discomfort.

Omega-3 Fatty Acids:

Sources: Found in fatty fish (salmon, mackerel), flaxseeds, chia seeds, and walnuts.

Benefits: Omega-3 fatty acids have anti-inflammatory properties, aiding in the management of conditions like rheumatoid arthritis and inflammatory bowel diseases.

Capsaicin (Chili Peppers):

Active Compound: Capsaicin is responsible for the spicy heat in chili peppers.

Usage: Topical capsaicin creams can be applied to the skin.

Benefits: Capsaicin is known for its analgesic properties, providing relief from conditions like osteoarthritis and neuropathic pain.

Arnica:

Derived from: Arnica montana, a perennial flower.

Usage: Arnica can be applied topically in the form of creams or gels.

Benefits: Traditionally used to reduce bruising, swelling, and inflammation associated with injuries.

Boswellia (Frankincense):

Active Compounds: Boswellic acids possess anti-inflammatory properties.

Usage: Available as a supplement or in topical forms.

Benefits: Boswellia has been studied for its potential in reducing symptoms of osteoarthritis and inflammatory bowel diseases.

Willow Bark:

Active Ingredient: Salicin, a natural compound similar to aspirin.

Usage: Willow bark supplements are available, or it can be consumed as a tea.

Benefits: Willow bark may help alleviate pain and inflammation, especially in conditions like osteoarthritis.

Lavender Essential Oil:

Usage: Inhaling lavender oil or diluting it for topical application.

Benefits: Lavender oil is known for its calming and analgesic effects, providing relief from headaches, migraines, and muscle tension.

While these natural remedies may offer relief for pain and inflammation, it's crucial to consult with a healthcare professional before incorporating them into your routine, especially if you have pre-existing medical conditions or are taking other medications. Additionally, maintaining a healthy lifestyle through proper diet, regular exercise, and stress management can contribute to overall well-being and further enhance the effectiveness of these natural remedies.

Herbal Solutions for Respiratory Issues

Respiratory issues can affect people of all ages, causing discomfort and disruptions to daily life. While conventional medicine offers effective treatments, many individuals seek natural remedies to complement their healthcare routine. Herbal solutions have been used for centuries to address various respiratory conditions, providing relief and supporting overall respiratory health. In this article, we explore some natural remedies for common respiratory issues.

Eucalyptus:

Background: Eucalyptus has been recognized for its respiratory benefits due to its active compound, cineole, which has anti-inflammatory and decongestant properties.

Application: Inhaling eucalyptus oil vapors through steam inhalation can help relieve nasal congestion and ease respiratory discomfort.

Peppermint:

Background: Peppermint contains menthol, a natural compound known for its ability to relax the muscles of the respiratory tract, promoting easier breathing.

Application: Peppermint tea or inhaling the scent of peppermint oil may alleviate symptoms like coughing and throat irritation.

Ginger:

Background: Ginger has anti-inflammatory properties and is known for its ability to soothe sore throats and reduce inflammation in the respiratory system.

Application: Drinking ginger tea or adding fresh ginger to meals can provide relief from respiratory discomfort.

Thyme:

Background: Thyme contains compounds with antimicrobial and expectorant properties, making it a valuable herb for respiratory health.

Application: Thyme tea or inhaling thyme-infused steam can help relieve respiratory congestion and support the body's natural defenses.

Licorice Root:

Background: Licorice root has been used in traditional medicine to soothe irritated throats and reduce inflammation in the respiratory system.

Application: Consuming licorice tea or incorporating licorice root supplements into your routine may offer relief from respiratory symptoms.

Turmeric:

Background: Curcumin, the active compound in turmeric, has anti-inflammatory and antioxidant properties that may benefit respiratory health.

Application: Adding turmeric to meals or consuming turmeric tea may help alleviate inflammation in the respiratory tract.

Garlic:

Background: Garlic is renowned for its antimicrobial properties, making it a natural remedy for respiratory infections.

Application: Incorporating raw or cooked garlic into your diet can support immune function and help combat respiratory infections.

Oregano:

Background: Oregano contains compounds like carvacrol with antimicrobial properties, making it effective against respiratory infections.

Application: Oregano oil or oregano tea can be used to alleviate symptoms of respiratory issues and boost overall respiratory health.

While these herbal remedies can provide relief for common respiratory conditions, it's essential to consult with a healthcare professional before incorporating them into your routine, especially if you are on medication or have underlying health conditions. Additionally, maintaining a healthy lifestyle, staying hydrated, and practicing good respiratory hygiene can further contribute to overall respiratory well-being.

Managing Digestive Problems With Natural Approaches

Digestive problems can significantly impact our daily lives, causing discomfort and disrupting our routines. While over-the-counter medications are readily available, many individuals seek natural remedies to address digestive issues. In this article, we'll explore natural approaches for managing common digestive problems.

Peppermint Oil for Indigestion:

Peppermint oil has long been recognized for its ability to alleviate indigestion symptoms. It helps relax the muscles of the gastrointestinal tract, reducing spasms and discomfort. Consuming peppermint tea or taking peppermint oil capsules before meals may provide relief from indigestion.

Ginger for Nausea:

Ginger has anti-inflammatory properties that make it an effective remedy for nausea and vomiting. Ginger tea or ginger capsules can be consumed to ease nausea associated with digestive issues. Additionally, chewing on a small piece of fresh ginger may provide quick relief.

Probiotics for Gut Health:

Probiotics are beneficial bacteria that promote a healthy balance of microorganisms in the gut. They can be found in fermented foods like yogurt, kefir, sauerkraut, and kimchi. Regular consumption of these probiotic-rich foods can enhance gut health and alleviate symptoms of bloating and irregular bowel movements.

Aloe Vera for Irritable Bowel Syndrome (IBS):

Aloe vera has anti-inflammatory properties and is known for its soothing effects on the digestive tract. It may be particularly helpful for individuals with irritable bowel syndrome (IBS). Consuming aloe vera juice in moderation can help reduce inflammation and provide relief from IBS symptoms.

Chamomile Tea for Gas and Bloating:

Chamomile tea has been traditionally used to ease digestive discomfort, including gas and bloating. It possesses anti-inflammatory and muscle-relaxant properties that can help soothe the digestive tract. Drinking chamomile tea after meals may aid in preventing or reducing gas and bloating.

Fiber-Rich Foods for Constipation:

A diet rich in fiber helps promote regular bowel movements and prevents constipation. Foods such as whole grains, fruits, vegetables, and legumes are excellent sources of dietary fiber. Increasing fiber intake gradually and staying hydrated can contribute to a healthy digestive system.

Fennel Seeds for Acid Reflux:

Fennel seeds have been used for centuries to alleviate symptoms of acid reflux. Chewing on a small handful of fennel seeds after meals can help reduce acidity and promote better digestion. Additionally, fennel tea may be a soothing option for those experiencing acid reflux.

Managing digestive problems with natural approaches involves incorporating wholesome remedies into your daily routine. While these natural remedies can be effective for many individuals, it's essential to consult with a healthcare professional if digestive issues persist or worsen. Maintaining a healthy lifestyle, including a balanced diet, regular exercise, and stress management, can also contribute to overall digestive well-being.

CHAPTER 5: ADVANCED NATURAL MEDICINE TECHNIQUES

Crafting Herbal Tinctures and Extracts

n the realm of natural medicine, herbal tinctures and extracts stand out as powerful remedies, offering a concentrated and convenient way to harness the healing properties of plants. Crafting these botanical wonders requires a blend of art and science, as practitioners draw upon ancient wisdom and modern techniques to create potent elixirs. This article delves into the world of advanced natural medicine techniques, exploring the art of crafting herbal tinctures and extracts for enhanced therapeutic benefits.

Understanding Herbal Tinctures and Extracts:

Herbal tinctures and extracts are liquid preparations derived from medicinal plants, capturing their active compounds in a concentrated form. Tinctures are typically alcohol-based, while extracts can use various solvents such as glycerin or vinegar. These methods allow for the extraction of a broad spectrum of bioactive compounds, including alkaloids, flavonoids, and essential oils.

Choosing High-Quality Herbs:

The foundation of any potent herbal remedy lies in the quality of the herbs used. Selecting organically grown, ethically harvested, and properly identified herbs ensures that the resulting tinctures and extracts are rich in therapeutic compounds. The choice of fresh or dried herbs also influences the final product, with each offering unique advantages.

Advanced Extraction Techniques:

Cold Maceration:

This technique involves steeping herbs in a solvent (usually alcohol) for an extended period without applying heat. Cold maceration preserves delicate compounds that can be destroyed by heat, resulting in a more nuanced and effective tincture.

Heat-Assisted Extraction:

For certain herbs with tougher cell walls, gentle heat can be applied during the extraction process. This helps break down the plant material, facilitating the release of active constituents. However, care must be taken to avoid excessive heat, which may compromise the quality of the final product.

Dual-Extraction Method:

Combining both water and alcohol extractions, this method is particularly effective for mushrooms and other plant materials that contain water-soluble and alcohol-soluble compounds. The resulting tincture showcases a broader spectrum of therapeutic benefits.

Spagyric Tinctures:

Rooted in alchemical traditions, spagyric tinctures involve not only extracting the soluble constituents but also incorporating the mineral salts and ash from the plant. This holistic approach is believed to enhance the overall therapeutic potency of the tincture.

Quality Control and Standardization:

Advanced natural medicine techniques include rigorous quality control measures and standardization processes. Practitioners may use analytical tools such as high-performance liquid chromatography (HPLC) to quantify specific compounds, ensuring consistency and potency across batches.

Crafting advanced herbal tinctures and extracts is a harmonious blend of ancient wisdom and modern science. By understanding the nuances of extraction techniques, choosing high-quality herbs, and implementing quality control measures, practitioners can unlock the full potential of these natural remedies. Whether used for immune support, stress relief, or addressing specific health concerns, advanced natural medicine techniques empower individuals to harness the healing power of plants in a concentrated and accessible form.

Exploring Alternative Healing Practices

:In recent years, there has been a growing interest in alternative healing practices that harness the power of nature to promote well-being and address health concerns. Advanced Natural Medicine Techniques go beyond conventional approaches, tapping into ancient wisdom and innovative methodologies to achieve holistic healing. In this article, we delve into the fascinating realm of advanced natural medicine, exploring techniques that blend traditional knowledge with cutting-edge science.

Herbal Medicine and Adaptogens:

Herbal medicine has been a cornerstone of natural healing for centuries. Advanced natural medicine takes it a step further by incorporating adaptogens—herbs that help the body adapt to stressors and restore balance. Plants like ashwagandha, rhodiola, and holy basil are revered for their adaptogenic properties, supporting the body's resilience against physical and mental stress.

Functional Nutrition and Nutraceuticals:

The field of functional nutrition focuses on the therapeutic use of food and nutrients to address specific health issues. Advanced natural medicine embraces this approach by tailoring dietary plans to individual needs. Nutraceuticals, which are nutrient-rich compounds with medicinal properties, are also gaining prominence. From curcumin to omega-3 fatty acids, these substances play a crucial role in supporting overall health.

Energy Medicine:

Energy medicine explores the subtle energy fields that surround and permeate the human body. Techniques such as acupuncture, Reiki, and Qi Gong are integral to advanced natural medicine. These practices aim to balance the body's energy, promoting physical, emotional, and spiritual well-being. By addressing the flow of vital energy, practitioners believe they can influence the body's ability to heal itself.

Biofeedback and Mind-Body Medicine:

Advanced natural medicine incorporates biofeedback and mind-body techniques to tap into the mind's influence on physical health. Biofeedback allows individuals to gain awareness and control over physiological functions, such as heart rate and muscle tension. Mind-body practices like meditation, mindfulness, and yoga are embraced for their ability to reduce stress, enhance mental clarity, and promote healing.

Environmental Medicine:

Acknowledging the impact of the environment on health, advanced natural medicine explores environmental medicine as a proactive approach to wellness. This includes addressing factors like air and water quality, electromagnetic fields, and toxins in daily life. By minimizing environmental stressors, individuals aim to create a healing environment conducive to optimal health.

Integrative Therapies:

Advanced natural medicine often integrates various healing modalities to create comprehensive treatment plans. Integrative medicine combines conventional and alternative approaches, considering the whole person rather than focusing solely on symptoms. This collaborative approach may include consultations with naturopathic doctors, holistic nutritionists, and other healthcare professionals.

As interest in holistic well-being continues to grow, advanced natural medicine techniques provide a bridge between traditional wisdom and modern science. By exploring alternative healing practices, individuals can embark on a journey toward optimal health, harnessing the power of nature to promote balance and vitality. Whether incorporating adaptogens, engaging in energy medicine, or embracing integrative therapies, the advanced natural medicine landscape offers a diverse and evolving path to wellness.

Integrating Natural Medicine into Long-Term Survival Strategies

In an era dominated by modern medicine, the resurgence of interest in natural and holistic healing methods is gaining momentum. Advanced natural medicine techniques offer a unique approach to health and well-being by harnessing the power of nature's remedies. In the context of long-term survival strategies, the integration of these techniques becomes even more crucial, as they provide sustainable and self-reliant solutions for maintaining optimal health.

Herbalism and Medicinal Plants:

One of the foundational pillars of advanced natural medicine is herbalism. Medicinal plants have been used for centuries by various cultures for their healing properties. In long-term survival scenarios, understanding the identification, cultivation, and application of medicinal plants becomes essential. From immune-boosting herbs like echinacea to pain-relieving plants like arnica, herbalism provides a vast array of options for holistic health maintenance.

Adaptogenic Herbs and Stress Management:
Adaptogens are a class of herbs that help the body adapt to stressors, both physical and mental. Long-term survival situations can be mentally and emotionally taxing, making adaptogens invaluable. Herbs such as ashwagandha, rhodiola, and holy basil are known for their ability to modulate the body's stress response, promoting resilience and overall well-being.

Holistic Nutrition:

In a survival context, proper nutrition is paramount for sustaining energy levels and maintaining overall health. Advanced natural medicine emphasizes the importance of whole foods, focusing on nutrient-dense options. Integrating superfoods, fermented foods, and a variety of organic produce ensures a well-rounded and balanced diet that supports the body's natural healing processes.

Aromatherapy and Essential Oils:

Aromatherapy harnesses the therapeutic properties of essential oils to enhance physical, emotional, and mental well-being. Essential oils such as lavender, peppermint, and tea tree oil have antimicrobial properties, making them valuable in a survival setting. Additionally, aromatherapy can play a crucial role in managing stress, anxiety, and promoting better sleep – vital aspects of long-term survival.

Holistic Practices:

Advanced natural medicine extends beyond physical remedies to encompass holistic practices that address the mind-body connection. Techniques like acupuncture, yoga, meditation, and mindfulness contribute to overall well-being by promoting relaxation, reducing stress, and enhancing the body's natural healing mechanisms.

DIY Remedies and First Aid:

In a survival scenario, access to conventional medical care may be limited. Knowing how to create simple, effective remedies from natural ingredients becomes invaluable. From herbal poultices to natural antiseptics, acquiring basic first aid skills using natural elements can be a lifesaver.

Incorporating advanced natural medicine techniques into long-term survival strategies provides a sustainable and self-sufficient approach to health and well-being. By tapping into the healing power of nature through herbalism, adaptogens, holistic nutrition, aromatherapy, holistic practices, and DIY remedies, individuals can empower themselves with the knowledge and skills needed for a resilient and healthy life. As we navigate an uncertain future, embracing these advanced natural medicine techniques becomes a holistic and proactive approach to safeguarding our well-being.

CONCLUSION

In conclusion, "Prepper's Survival Natural Medicine" stands as a crucial and comprehensive guide in the realm of emergency preparedness, providing an invaluable resource for individuals navigating situations where traditional medical assistance is unavailable. Authored with acute insight into the challenges of survival in adverse conditions, this handbook meticulously combines the principles of prepping with an extensive understanding of natural medicine.

The book serves as a beacon of empowerment, equipping readers with the knowledge and skills necessary to address medical emergencies when expert assistance is beyond reach. The emphasis on first aid, life-saving herbs, and natural remedies sets it apart, acknowledging the practical reality that, in certain scenarios, relying solely on conventional medical practices may not be feasible.

One of the book's notable strengths lies in its meticulous approach to first aid, offering a detailed exploration of fundamental techniques that can mean the difference between life and death in critical situations. The guidance provided covers a spectrum of emergencies, from minor injuries to more severe incidents, ensuring that readers are well-prepared to handle diverse medical challenges.

The incorporation of life-saving herbs and natural remedies further enriches the book's utility. The author demonstrates a profound understanding of the healing properties inherent in nature, providing readers with a toolkit of botanical solutions. This emphasis on natural alternatives not only aligns with the prepper ethos of self-sufficiency but also acknowledges the potential scarcity of pharmaceutical resources in a survival scenario.

In addition to its practical advice, "Prepper's Survival Natural Medicine" excels in fostering a mindset of preparedness. The book goes beyond mere instruction, instilling a sense of responsibility and self-reliance in its readers. By presenting a comprehensive approach that encompasses both physical and mental preparedness, it empowers individuals to face emergencies with confidence and competence.

Furthermore, the book acknowledges the reality of a world where professional medical assistance may not be readily available. In doing so, it provides an essential bridge between conventional first aid manuals and the unique challenges posed by survival scenarios. It bridges the gap between theory and practice, ensuring that readers are not only informed but also capable of applying their knowledge effectively.

As we navigate an ever-changing world with unpredictable challenges, "Prepper's Survival Natural Medicine" stands as a beacon of wisdom, offering a roadmap for those who understand the importance of being prepared for the unexpected. Its holistic approach, blending emergency preparedness with natural medicine, positions it as an indispensable guide for anyone committed to safeguarding their well-being and that of their loved ones in times of crisis. This book is not just a manual; it's a testament to the resilience of the human spirit and the resourcefulness that can be cultivated when armed with the right knowledge. "Prepper's Survival Natural Medicine" is an investment in one's ability to adapt, survive, and thrive in the face of adversity.